STROKE RECOVERY
COOKBOOK FOR SENIORS

Quick and easy recipes to improve stability,heal paralysis aid stroke rehabilitation

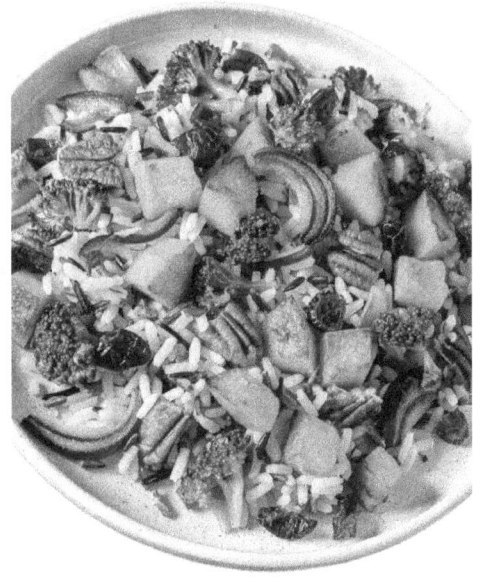

Dr. Malvin Harison

TABLE OF CONTENT

Introduction

Step into the kitchen, where healing meets flavor in "STROKE RECOVERY COOKBOOK." This isn't just a cookbook; it's a culinary companion tailored for seniors rediscovering the joy of eating post-stroke. Within these pages, we've crafted a collection of delightful recipes, each one a harmony of nutrition and pleasure.

From comforting classics to innovative dishes, we've curated a selection designed not only to tantalize taste buds but also to kindle a renewed enthusiasm for life. Each recipe is a brushstroke on the canvas of your well-being. A reminder that the kitchen is more than just a room; it's a sanctuary where healing begins, and the joy of cooking becomes a celebration of life.

So, let's embark on this culinary adventure together, savoring each step toward renewal with every delicious recipe.

Understand Stroke

A stroke, often referred to as a brain attack, occurs when the blood supply to a part of the brain is obstructed or when a blood vessel in the brain ruptures.

In either scenario, sections of the brain sustain damage or undergo cell death. A stroke has the potential to result in persistent brain damage, long-term disability, or even fatality. The brain plays a crucial role in controlling movements, storing memories, and serving as the origin of thoughts, emotions, and language. Additionally, it regulates various bodily functions such as breathing and digestion.

For optimal functionality, the brain requires a constant supply of oxygen. Oxygen-rich blood is transported to all areas of the brain through the arteries. If there's an impediment to the blood flow, brain cells begin to die within minutes due to the lack of oxygen, leading to the occurrence of a stroke.

The Significance of Taking the Right Diet

Maintaining a well-balanced and nutritious diet is crucial for stroke management in seniors.
Here are key reasons highlighting the importance of the right diet:

1. Promotes Brain Health: A diet rich in antioxidants, omega-3 fatty acids, and vitamins supports overall brain health, helping to prevent further damage and support recovery.

2. Manages Blood Pressure: High blood pressure is a significant risk factor for strokes. A diet low in sodium and high in potassium, such as the DASH (Dietary Approaches to Stop Hypertension) diet, can help regulate blood pressure and reduce the risk of recurrent strokes.

3. Controls Cholesterol Levels: A heart-healthy diet that includes fiber-rich foods, whole grains, and healthy fats helps manage cholesterol levels, reducing the risk of atherosclerosis and subsequent strokes.

4. Supports Weight Management: Maintaining a healthy weight is essential for seniors. A well-balanced diet, coupled with regular physical activity, contributes to weight management and overall well-being.

5. Manages Diabetes: For seniors with diabetes, controlling blood sugar levels is crucial. A diet that controls carbohydrate intake and includes whole, nutrient-dense foods can help manage diabetes and reduce the risk of complications like stroke.

6. Aids in Rehabilitation: Nutrient-dense foods provide the energy and essential nutrients needed for the rehabilitation process after a stroke. Adequate protein intake supports muscle strength and recovery.

7. Reduces Inflammation: An anti-inflammatory diet, including fruits, vegetables, and fatty fish, can help reduce inflammation in the body, which is linked to various chronic conditions, including stroke.

8. Enhances Digestive Health: A diet rich in fiber from fruits, vegetables, and whole grains supports digestive health, preventing constipation and promoting a healthy gut microbiome.

9. Ensures Hydration: Staying well-hydrated is essential for overall health. Seniors should maintain an adequate fluid intake, which is crucial for optimal brain function and can also help prevent complications like urinary tract infections.

10. Addresses Nutrient Deficiencies: Seniors may be at a higher risk of nutrient deficiencies. A well-planned diet ensures an adequate intake of essential nutrients, including vitamins and minerals crucial for overall health and recovery.

Complications if the right diet is not taken

Failure to adopt a proper diet following a stroke can lead to various complications, hindering recovery and potentially increasing the risk of further health issues. Here are some potential complications associated with not following an appropriate diet after a stroke:

1. Increased Risk of Recurrent Stroke: Poor dietary choices can contribute to persistent risk factors such as high blood pressure, high cholesterol, and diabetes, increasing the likelihood of experiencing another stroke.

2. Worsening of Cardiovascular Health: Unhealthy eating habits may lead to elevated blood pressure and cholesterol levels, putting additional strain on the cardiovascular system and increasing the risk of heart-related complications.

3. Impaired Cognitive Function: Inadequate nutrition may negatively impact cognitive function and memory, hindering the recovery process and diminishing the overall quality of life for stroke survivors.

4. Reduced Energy Levels and Fatigue: A lack of essential nutrients can lead to fatigue and decreased energy levels, making it challenging for individuals to engage in necessary rehabilitation exercises and daily activities.

5. Weakened Immune System: Poor nutrition can compromise the immune system, making individuals more susceptible to infections and other health issues, which can impede recovery.

6. Muscle Weakness and Loss of Mobility: Insufficient protein intake and inadequate nutrition can contribute to muscle weakness and loss of mobility, hindering rehabilitation efforts and overall physical recovery.

7. Increased Risk of Complications: Malnutrition or deficiencies in essential nutrients can lead to complications such as pressure ulcers, infections, and delayed wound healing, particularly in seniors who may already have compromised health.

8. Nutrient Deficiencies and Bone Health Issues: Inadequate intake of calcium and vitamin D, essential for bone health, can lead to bone density issues, increasing the risk of fractures and complications in the aging population.

9. Digestive Problems: Poor dietary choices, such as insufficient fiber intake, can lead to digestive issues like constipation, affecting overall gastrointestinal health.

10. Mental Health Challenges: Lack of proper nutrition may contribute to mood swings, depression, and anxiety, impacting mental health and well-being during the recovery process.

Chapter 1: Delicious Breakfast Recipes

Here are 10 nutrient-rich and stroke recovery-friendly breakfast recipes for seniors;

1. Berry Blast Smoothie Bowl

Ingredients
- 1 cup of different berries (blueberries, strawberries, raspberries)
- 1 banana
- 1/2 cup Greek yogurt
- 1 tablespoon chia seeds
- 1 tablespoon honey
- 1/2 cup almond milk

Preparation
1. Blend berries, banana, Greek yogurt, chia seeds, honey, and almond milk until smooth.
2. Pour into a bowl and top with additional berries, sliced banana, and a sprinkle of chia seeds.

Servings: 1

Nutritional Value (approx.): 350 calories, 10g protein, 8g fiber, 25g sugar
Cooking Time: 5 minutes

2. Avocado and Smoked Salmon Toast

Ingredients
- 1 slice whole-grain bread
- 1/2 avocado, mashed
- 2 oz smoked salmon
- 1 teaspoon lemon juice
- Fresh dill for garnish

Preparation
1. Toast the bread to your liking.
2. Spread mashed avocado on the toast, top with smoked salmon, and drizzle with lemon juice.
3. Garnish with fresh dill.

Servings: 1

Nutritional Value (approx.): 300 calories, 15g protein, 8g fiber, 2g sugar
Cooking Time: 5 minutes

3. Quinoa Breakfast Bowl

Ingredients
- 1/2 cup cooked quinoa
- 1/4 cup Greek yogurt
- 1/4 cup fresh mango, diced
- 1 tablespoon pumpkin seeds
- Drizzle of honey

Preparation
1. In a bowl, layer cooked quinoa, Greek yogurt, and diced mango.
2. Top with pumpkin seeds and drizzle with honey.

Servings: 1

Nutritional Value (approx.): 280 calories, 10g protein, 5g fiber, 12g sugar

Cooking Time: 10 minutes (if quinoa is pre-cooked)

4. Spinach and Feta Omelet

Ingredients
- 2 large eggs
- Handful of fresh spinach
- 2 tablespoons crumbled feta cheese
- 1 teaspoon olive oil

- Salt and pepper to taste

Preparation

1. Whisk eggs in a bowl and season with salt and pepper.

2. Heat olive oil in a pan, add spinach, and sauté until wilted.

3. Pour whisked eggs over the spinach, add feta, and cook until set. Fold in half before serving.

Servings: 1

Nutritional Value (approx.): 250 calories, 18g protein, 2g fiber, 1g sugar

Cooking Time: 8 minutes

5. Chia Seed Pudding with Berries

Ingredients

- 2 tablespoons chia seeds
- 1/2 cup almond milk
- 1/2 teaspoon vanilla extract
- 1/2 cup mixed berries

Preparation

1. Combine chia seeds, almond milk, and vanilla extract in a bowl. Refrigerate for about 2 hours, preferably overnight.

2. Top with mixed berries before serving.

Servings: 1

Nutritional Value (approx.): 220 calories, 6g protein, 10g fiber, 8g sugar

Cooking Time: 5 minutes (plus refrigeration time)

6. Whole Grain Pancakes with Greek Yogurt

Ingredients
- 1/2 cup whole wheat flour
- 1/2 teaspoon baking powder
- 1/2 cup almond milk
- 1 egg
- 1 tablespoon maple syrup
- 1/2 cup Greek yogurt
- Fresh fruit for topping

Preparation

1. In a bowl, whisk together flour, baking powder, almond milk, egg, and maple syrup until smooth.

2. Pour batter onto a hot, greased pan to make small pancakes.

Cook till bubbles are forming, then turn and cook the other side.

3. Top with Greek yogurt and fresh fruit.

Servings: 2-3

Nutritional Value (approx. per serving): 180 calories, 8g protein, 3g fiber, 8g sugar

Cooking Time: 15 minutes

7. Sweet Potato and Kale Breakfast Hash

Ingredients

- 1 medium sweet potato, diced
- Handful of kale, chopped
- 1 egg
- 1 teaspoon olive oil
- Salt and pepper to taste

Preparation

1. Heat olive oil in a pan, add sweet potatoes, and cook until slightly tender.

2. Add chopped kale and cook until wilted.

3. Create a well in the hash and crack an egg into it. Cover and cook till the egg is done.

Servings: 1
Nutritional Value (approx.): 280 calories, 10g protein, 6g fiber, 5g sugar
Cooking Time: 15 minutes

8. Yogurt Parfait with Nuts and Berries

Ingredients
- 1 cup plain Greek yogurt
- 1/4 cup granola
- 1/4 cup of different nuts (almonds, walnuts)
- 1/2 cup of different berries
- Drizzle of honey

Preparation
1. In a glass, layer Greek yogurt, granola, mixed nuts, and berries.
2. Drizzle with honey before serving.

Servings: 1
Nutritional Value (approx.): 320 calories, 20g protein, 5g fiber, 12g sugar
Cooking Time: 5 minutes

9. Oatmeal with Banana and Almond Butter

Ingredients
- 1/2 cup old-fashioned oats
- 1 cup almond milk
- 1 banana, sliced
- 1 tablespoon almond butter
- Cinnamon for flavor

Preparation
1. Cook oats with almond milk until creamy.
2. Add banana slices, almond butter, and a spray of cinnamon.

Servings: 1

Nutritional Value (approx.): 280 calories, 8g protein, 6g fiber, 10g sugar

Cooking Time: 10 minutes

10. Salmon and Vegetable Breakfast Wrap

Ingredients
- 1 whole-grain wrap
- 2 oz smoked salmon

- 1/4 avocado, sliced
- Handful of spinach leaves
- 1 teaspoon Greek yogurt (as a spread)

Preparation

1. Spread Greek yogurt on the whole-grain wrap.

2. Layer with smoked salmon, sliced avocado, and spinach leaves.

3. Roll up the wrap and slice if desired.

Servings: 1

Nutritional Value (approx.): 320 calories, 20g protein, 5g fiber, 2g sugar

Cooking Time: 5 minutes

Chapter 2: Satisfying Lunch

Here are 10 nutrient-rich and stroke recovery-friendly lunch recipes for seniors;

1. Grilled Salmon with Quinoa and Vegetables

Ingredients
- 1 salmon filet
- 1/2 cup cooked quinoa
- Mixed vegetables (e.g., broccoli, bell peppers)
- 1 tablespoon olive oil
- Lemon slices for garnish

Preparation
1. Season the salmon with salt and pepper and grill until cooked.
2. Sauté mixed vegetables in olive oil until tender.
3. Serve the grilled salmon over a bed of quinoa with sautéed vegetables. Garnish with lemon slices.

Servings: 1
Nutritional Value (approx.): 400 calories, 25g protein, 10g fiber, 5g sugar
Cooking Time: 20 minutes

2. Turkey and Avocado Wrap with Quinoa Salad

Ingredients
- 4 oz sliced turkey breast
- 1 whole-grain wrap
- 1/2 avocado, sliced
- Mixed greens
- 1/2 cup quinoa salad (quinoa, cherry tomatoes, cucumber, feta)

Preparation
1. Layer turkey slices, avocado, and mixed greens on the wrap.
2. Roll up the wrap and serve with a side of quinoa salad.

Servings: 1
Nutritional Value (approx.): 380 calories, 20g protein, 8g fiber, 5g sugar
Cooking Time: 15 minutes

3. Chicken Vegetable Stir-Fry

Ingredients
- 4 oz grilled chicken breast, sliced
- Mixed stir-fry vegetables (bell peppers, broccoli, carrots)
- 1 cup cooked brown rice
- 1 tablespoon low-sodium soy sauce
- 1 teaspoon sesame oil

Preparation
1. Stir-fry chicken slices and mixed vegetables in sesame oil.
2. Add cooked brown rice and soy sauce, tossing until well combined.

Servings: 1
Nutritional Value (approx.): 380 calories, 25g protein, 8g fiber, 4g sugar
Cooking Time: 15 minutes

4. Quinoa and Chickpea Salad

Ingredients
- 1/2 cup cooked quinoa
- 1/2 cup canned chickpeas, drained and rinsed

- Cherry tomatoes, halved
- Cucumber, diced
- Fresh parsley, chopped
- 1 tablespoon tahini
- Juice of 1 lemon

Preparation

1. Combine quinoa, chickpeas, cherry tomatoes, cucumber, and parsley in a bowl.

2. Whisk together tahini and lemon juice to create the dressing. Drizzle over the salad.

Servings: 1

Nutritional Value (approx.): 320 calories, 12g protein, 8g fiber, 4g sugar

Cooking Time: 10 minutes

5. Sweet Potato and Lentil Soup

Ingredients

- 1 medium sweet potato, diced
- 1/2 cup lentils
- 1 carrot, sliced
- 1 onion, chopped
- 2 cloves garlic, minced

- Vegetable broth
- 1 teaspoon turmeric
- Salt and pepper to taste

Preparation

1. Sauté onion and garlic in a pot until softened.

2. Add sweet potato, lentils, carrot, turmeric, salt, and pepper. Cover with vegetable broth and simmer until vegetables are tender.

Servings: 2

Nutritional Value (approx. per serving): 250 calories, 10g protein, 8g fiber, 5g sugar

Cooking Time: 30 minutes

6. Mango and Shrimp Salad

Ingredients

- 4 oz cooked shrimp, peeled and deveined
- Mixed salad greens
- 1/2 mango, diced
- Cherry tomatoes, halved
- 1/4 cup feta cheese

- Olive oil and balsamic vinegar for dressing

Preparation

1. Toss shrimp, salad greens, mango, cherry tomatoes, and feta in a bowl.

2. Drizzle with olive oil and balsamic vinegar.

Servings: 1

Nutritional Value (approx.): 320 calories, 20g protein, 6g fiber, 8g sugar

Cooking Time: 15 minutes

7. Egg and Vegetable Frittata

Ingredients

- 2 eggs
- Bell peppers, spinach, and cherry tomatoes (or vegetables of choice)
- 1 tablespoon feta cheese
- Salt and pepper to taste

Preparation

1. Whisk eggs and season with salt and pepper.
2. Sauté vegetables in an oven-safe pan, then pour whisked eggs over them.
3. Sprinkle with feta cheese and bake until the eggs are set.

Servings: 1

Nutritional Value (approx.): 280 calories, 15g protein, 4g fiber, 3g sugar

Cooking Time: 20 minutes

8. Salmon and Asparagus Foil Pack

Ingredients

- 1 salmon filet
- Asparagus spears
- Lemon slices

- Fresh dill
- Olive oil
- Salt and pepper to taste

Preparation

1. Place salmon on a piece of foil, surround with asparagus, and top with lemon slices and fresh dill.

2. Drizzle with olive oil, season with salt and pepper, and fold the foil to create a pack.

3. Bake until salmon is cooked through.

Servings: 1

Nutritional Value (approx.): 350 calories, 25g protein, 8g fiber, 2g sugar

Cooking Time: 20 minutes

9. Chickpea and Spinach Stew

Ingredients

- 1 can chickpeas, drained and rinsed
- 2 cups fresh spinach
- 1 onion, chopped
- 2 cloves garlic, minced
- 1 can diced tomatoes
- Vegetable broth
- 1 teaspoon cumin

- Salt and pepper to taste

Preparation

1. Sauté onion and garlic until softened.

2. Add chickpeas, spinach, diced tomatoes, cumin, salt, and pepper. Cover with vegetable broth and simmer until flavors meld.

Servings: 2

Nutritional Value (approx. per serving): 280 calories, 12g protein, 8g fiber, 5g sugar

Cooking Time: 25 minutes

10. Greek Chicken Salad Bowl

Ingredients

- 4 oz grilled chicken breast, sliced
- Mixed salad greens
- Cherry tomatoes, halved
- Cucumber, diced
- Kalamata olives
- Feta cheese
- Lemon juice

Preparation

1. Assemble salad greens, cherry tomatoes, cucumber, olives, and feta in a bowl.

2. Top with grilled chicken slices and drizzle with lemon juice.

Servings: 1

Nutritional Value (approx.): 350 calories, 25g protein, 6g fiber, 4g sugar

Cooking Time: 15 minutes

Chapter 3: Nutritious Dinner

Here are 10 nutrient-rich and stroke recovery-friendly dinner recipes for seniors:

1. Baked Herb-Crusted Cod

Ingredients

- 1 cod filet
- 1 tablespoon olive oil
- Fresh herbs (such as parsley, thyme)
- Mixed vegetables (e.g., carrots, Brussels sprouts)
- Salt and pepper to taste

Preparation

1. Coat cod with olive oil and sprinkle with fresh herbs, salt, and pepper.
2. Roast cod and mixed vegetables in the oven until the fish flakes easily.

Servings: 1

Nutritional Value (approx.): 300 calories, 25g protein, 8g fiber, 4g sugar

Cooking Time: 25 minutes

2. Vegetarian Quinoa-Stuffed Bell Peppers

Ingredients
- 2 bell peppers, halved
- 1/2 cup cooked quinoa
- Black beans, corn, tomatoes (as desired)
- 1/4 cup shredded cheese
- Taco seasoning
- Fresh cilantro for garnish

Preparation
1. Mix cooked quinoa with black beans, corn, tomatoes, taco seasoning, and cheese.
2. Stuff bell peppers with the quinoa mixture and bake until peppers are tender.

Servings: 2

Nutritional Value (approx. per serving): 250 calories, 12g protein, 6g fiber, 4g sugar

Cooking Time: 30 minutes

3. Lemon Garlic Chicken with Brown Rice and Broccoli

Ingredients

- 4 oz grilled chicken breast
- 1 cup cooked brown rice
- Steamed broccoli
- Zest and juice of 1 lemon
- Garlic powder, salt, and pepper to taste

Preparation

1. Season grilled chicken with lemon zest, lemon juice, garlic powder, salt, and pepper.
2. Serve over a bed of brown rice with steamed broccoli on the side.

Servings: 1

Nutritional Value (approx.): 350 calories, 30g protein, 6g fiber, 3g sugar

Cooking Time: 20 minutes

4. Salmon and Quinoa Patties

Ingredients

- 1 can canned salmon, drained
- 1/2 cup cooked quinoa
- 1 egg

- Chopped green onions
- Dill, salt, and pepper to taste
- Olive oil for cooking

Preparation

1. Mix salmon, cooked quinoa, egg, green onions, dill, salt, and pepper in a bowl.

2. Form into patties and cook in olive oil until golden brown.

Servings: 2

Nutritional Value (approx. per serving): 280 calories, 25g protein, 5g fiber, 1g sugar

Cooking Time: 15 minutes

5. Veggie-Packed Lentil Soup

Ingredients

- 1 cup lentils
- Carrots, celery, onions, and garlic (diced)
- Vegetable broth
- Spinach leaves
- Cumin, turmeric, salt, and pepper to taste

Preparation

1. Sauté carrots, celery, onions, and garlic until softened.
2. Add lentils, vegetable broth, cumin, turmeric, salt, and pepper. Simmer until lentils are tender.
3. Stir in spinach just before serving.

Servings: 4

Nutritional Value (approx. per serving): 200 calories, 12g protein, 8g fiber, 4g sugar

Cooking Time: 30 minutes

6. Eggplant and Chickpea Curry

Ingredients
- 1 medium eggplant, diced
- 1 can chickpeas, drained and rinsed
- 1 onion, chopped
- 2 cloves garlic, minced
- 1 can diced tomatoes
- Coconut milk
- Curry powder, cumin, salt, and pepper to taste

Preparation
1. Sauté eggplant, onion, and garlic until softened.

2. Add chickpeas, diced tomatoes, coconut milk, curry powder, cumin, salt, and pepper. Simmer until flavors meld.

Servings: 3

Nutritional Value (approx. per serving): 280 calories, 10g protein, 10g fiber, 6g sugar

Cooking Time: 25 minutes

7. Turkey and Vegetable Skewers with Quinoa

Ingredients
- 4 oz turkey breast, cubed
- Bell peppers, zucchini, cherry tomatoes
- Olive oil and lemon juice for marinade
- Quinoa, cooked
- Fresh herbs for garnish

Preparation

1. Marinate turkey and vegetables in a mix of olive oil and lemon juice.

2. Thread onto skewers and grill until turkey is cooked.

3. Serve over a bed of cooked quinoa, garnished with fresh herbs.

Servings: 2

Nutritional Value (approx. per serving): 300 calories, 20g protein, 6g fiber, 4g sugar
Cooking Time: 20 minutes

8. Mushroom and Spinach Stuffed Chicken Breast

Ingredients
- 2 chicken breasts
- 1 cup sliced mushrooms
- 1 cup fresh spinach
- Garlic, thyme, salt, and pepper to taste
- Olive oil for cooking

Preparation
1. Sauté mushrooms and spinach with garlic, thyme, salt, and pepper until wilted.
2. Cut a pocket in each chicken breast and stuff with the mushroom and spinach mixture.
3. Bake until chicken is cooked through.
Servings: 2
Nutritional Value (approx. per serving): 320 calories, 30g protein, 5g fiber, 2g sugar

Cooking Time: 25 minutes

9. Shrimp and Vegetable Stir-Fry with Brown Rice

Ingredients
- 4 oz shrimp, peeled and deveined
- Mixed stir-fry vegetables (broccoli, snap peas, carrots)
- 1 cup cooked brown rice
- Low-sodium soy sauce, ginger, garlic, and sesame oil for flavor

Preparation
1. Stir-fry shrimp and mixed vegetables in sesame oil, ginger, and garlic.
2. Add cooked brown rice and soy sauce, tossing until well combined.

Servings: 1

Nutritional Value (approx.): 320 calories, 20g protein, 8g fiber, 4g sugar

Cooking Time: 15 minutes

10. Caprese Quinoa Bowl

Ingredients

- 1/2 cup cooked quinoa
- Cherry tomatoes, halved
- Fresh mozzarella, diced
- Fresh basil leaves
- Balsamic glaze for drizzling
- Salt and pepper to taste

Preparation

1. In a bowl, combine cooked quinoa, cherry tomatoes, fresh mozzarella, and basil leaves.

2. Drizzle with balsamic glaze and season with salt and pepper.

Servings: 1

Nutritional Value (approx.): 300 calories, 15g protein, 5g fiber, 3g sugar

Cooking Time: 15 minutes

Chapter 4: Snacks and Dessert Recipes

Here are 10 nutrient-rich snacks and dessert recipes suitable for stroke recovery seniors;

1. Fruit and Nut Parfait

Ingredients
- 1 cup Greek yogurt
- Mixed berries (blueberries, strawberries)
- 1 tablespoon chopped almonds
- 1 tablespoon honey

Preparation
1. In a glass, layer Greek yogurt, mixed berries, and chopped almonds.
2. Drizzle with honey before serving.

Servings: 1

Nutritional Value (approx.): 250 calories, 15g protein, 5g fiber, 15g sugar

Preparation Time: 5 minutes

2. Avocado Chocolate Mousse

Ingredients
- 1 ripe avocado
- 2 tablespoons cocoa powder
- 2 tablespoons honey
- 1/2 teaspoon vanilla extract

Preparation
1. Blend avocado, cocoa powder, honey, and vanilla extract until smooth.
2. Chill in the refrigerator before serving.

Servings: 2

Nutritional Value (approx. per serving): 200 calories, 3g protein, 5g fiber, 15g sugar

Preparation Time: 10 minutes

3. Chia Seed and Mango Pudding

Ingredients
- 2 tablespoons chia seeds
- 1/2 cup almond milk
- 1/2 cup diced mango
- 1 teaspoon honey

Preparation

1. Combine chia seeds and almond milk. Refrigerate for at least 2 hours.

2. Top with diced mango and drizzle with honey.

Servings: 1

Nutritional Value (approx.): 220 calories, 5g protein, 8g fiber, 12g sugar

Preparation Time: 5 minutes (plus refrigeration time)

4. Whole Grain Banana Bread

Ingredients

- 2 ripe bananas, mashed
- 1/4 cup coconut oil
- 1/4 cup honey
- 1 teaspoon vanilla extract
- 1 cup whole wheat flour
- 1/2 teaspoon baking soda

Preparation

1. Mix mashed bananas, coconut oil, honey, and vanilla extract.

2. Stir in whole wheat flour and baking soda.

3. Bake in a preheated oven until a toothpick comes out clean.

Servings: 8
Nutritional Value (approx. per serving): 150 calories, 2g protein, 3g fiber, 12g sugar
Preparation Time: 30 minutes

5. Nut and Seed Energy Balls

Ingredients
- 1/2 cup mixed nuts (almonds, walnuts)
- 1/4 cup mixed seeds (flaxseeds, chia seeds)
- 2 tablespoons nut butter
- 1 tablespoon honey
- Desiccated coconut for rolling

Preparation
1. Blend nuts and seeds until finely ground.
2. Mix with nut butter and honey, then form into small balls.
3. Roll each ball in desiccated coconut.
Servings: 10
Nutritional Value (approx. per serving): 120 calories, 4g protein, 3g fiber, 6g sugar
Preparation Time: 15 minutes

6. Yogurt and Berry Popsicles

Ingredients
- 1 cup Greek yogurt
- Mixed berries (strawberries, blueberries)
- 1 tablespoon honey

Preparation
1. Mix Greek yogurt and honey.
2. Layer yogurt and mixed berries in popsicle molds.
3. Freeze until solid.

Servings: 4

Nutritional Value (approx. per serving): 80 calories, 4g protein, 2g fiber, 10g sugar

Preparation Time: 10 minutes (plus freezing time)

7. Apple and Almond Butter Sandwiches

Ingredients
- 1 apple, sliced
- Almond butter
- Cinnamon for sprinkling

Preparation

1. Spread almond butter on apple slices.

2. Create sandwiches and sprinkle with cinnamon.

Servings: 2

Nutritional Value (approx. per serving): 150 calories, 3g protein, 5g fiber, 10g sugar

Preparation Time: 5 minutes

8. Baked Cinnamon-Sweet Potato Fries

Ingredients

- 1 sweet potato, cut into fries
- 1 tablespoon coconut oil
- 1 teaspoon cinnamon
- Pinch of sea salt

Preparation

1. Toss sweet potato fries with melted coconut oil, cinnamon, and sea salt.

2. Bake until crispy in a preheated oven.

Servings: 2

Nutritional Value (approx. per serving): 120 calories, 2g protein, 4g fiber, 6g sugar

Preparation Time:.25 minutes

9. Peach and Berry Sorbet

Ingredients
- 2 cups frozen peaches
- 1/2 cup mixed berries
- 1 tablespoon honey
- Splash of water

Preparation
1. Blend frozen peaches, mixed berries, honey, and water until smooth.
2. Freeze for an additional 2 hours before serving.

Servings: 2

Nutritional Value (approx. per serving): 100 calories, 1g protein, 3g fiber, 18g sugar

Preparation Time: 10 minutes (plus freezing time)

10. Cottage Cheese with Pineapple and Mint

Ingredients

- 1/2 cup low-fat cottage cheese
- 1/2 cup diced pineapple
- Fresh mint leaves for garnish

Preparation

1. Mix cottage cheese with diced pineapple.

2. Garnish with fresh mint leaves before serving.

Servings: 1

Nutritional Value (approx.): 150 calories, 14g protein, 2g fiber, 10g sugar

Preparation Time: 5 minutes

Chapter 5:Bonus 1

7-days Meal plan

Here's a 7-day meal plan for stroke recovery seniors, incorporating a variety of nutrient-rich recipes for breakfast, lunch, dinner, and snacks;

Day 1

Breakfast: Nutrient-Packed Smoothie Bowl
Lunch: Grilled Salmon with Quinoa and Vegetables
Snack: Fruit and Nut Parfait
Dinner: Baked Herb-Crusted Cod with Roasted Vegetables

Day 2

Breakfast: Greek Yogurt
Lunch: Turkey and Avocado Wrap with Quinoa Salad
Snack: Avocado Chocolate Mousse

Dinner: Vegetarian Quinoa-Stuffed Bell Peppers

Day 3

Breakfast: Egg and Vegetable Frittata
Lunch: Chicken and Vegetable Stir-Fry with Brown Rice
Snack: Chia Seed and Mango Pudding
Dinner: Lemon Garlic Chicken with Brown Rice and Broccoli

Day 4

Breakfast: Cottage Cheese with Pineapple and Mint
Lunch: Quinoa and Chickpea Salad with Lemon-Tahini Dressing
Snack: Nut and Seed Energy Balls
Dinner: Salmon and Quinoa Patties

Day 5

Breakfast: Baked Cinnamon-Sweet Potato Fries
Lunch: Shrimp and Vegetable Stir-Fry with Brown Rice

Snack: Yogurt and Berry Popsicles
Dinner: Mushroom and Spinach Stuffed Chicken Breast

Day 6

Breakfast: Whole Grain Banana Bread
Lunch: Chickpea and Spinach Stew
Snack: Peach and Berry Sorbet
Dinner: Caprese Quinoa Bowl

Day 7

Breakfast: Apple and Almond Butter Sandwiches
Lunch: Greek Chicken Salad Bowl
Snack: Fruit and Nut Parfait
Dinner: Baked Herb-Crusted Cod with Roasted Vegetables

Chapter 6: Bonus 2

20 Juicing and Smoothie Recipes

Here are the 20 juicing and smoothie recipes for stroke recovery seniors:

1. Green Goddess Juice

Ingredients
- 1 cup kale
- 1 cucumber
- 1 green apple
- 1/2 lemon (peeled)
- 1-inch ginger

Instructions

1. Wash all ingredients thoroughly.

2. Cut them into smaller pieces for easier juicing.

3. Juice all the ingredients.

4. Stir well and serve immediately.

2. Heart-Healthy Red Juice

Ingredients

- 1 beet
- 1 cup berries (blueberries or strawberries)
- 1 carrot
- 1/2 lemon (peeled)

Instructions

1. Prepare and wash the ingredients.
2. Cut them into juicer-friendly pieces.
3. Juice the ingredients together.
4. Mix well and enjoy.

3. Anti-Inflammatory Turmeric Citrus Juice

Ingredients

- 2 oranges
- 1/2 lemon (peeled)
- 1-inch turmeric root
- 1 carrot

Instructions

1. Clean and chop all ingredients.
2. Juice them using a juicer.
3. Stir the juice and serve fresh.

4. Hydrating Cucumber Mint Juice

Ingredients
- 2 cucumbers
- Handful of mint leaves
- 1 green apple
- 1/2 lime (peeled)

Instructions
1. Wash and chop the ingredients.

2. Juice them together.

3. Add a squeeze of lime, stir, and serve.

5. Vitamin C Boost Juice

Ingredients
- 2 oranges
- 1 grapefruit
- 1 kiwi
- 1/2 lemon (peeled)

Instructions
1. Prepare the fruits and peel as needed.

2. Juice all the fruits together.

3. Mix well and serve immediately.

6. Berry Blast Smoothie

Ingredients
- 1 cup of different berries (strawberries, blueberries, raspberries)
- 1 banana
- 1/2 cup Greek yogurt
- 1 tablespoon chia seeds

Instructions
1. Add all ingredients in a blender.
2. Blend until smooth.
3. Pour into a glass and enjoy.

7. Creamy Avocado Spinach Smoothie

Ingredients
- 1/2 avocado
- Handful of spinach
- 1/2 banana
- 1/2 cup almond milk
- 1 tablespoon flax seeds

Instructions
1. Blend all ingredients until creamy.
2. Pour into a glass and serve.

8. Tropical Paradise Smoothie

Ingredients

- 1 cup pineapple chunks
- 1/2 mango
- 1/2 banana
- 1/2 cup coconut water
- 1 tablespoon hemp seeds

Instructions

1. Blend all ingredients until smooth.
2. Pour into a glass and serve.

9. Protein-Packed Peanut

Ingredients

- 1 banana
- 2 tablespoons peanut butter
- 1/2 cup Greek yogurt
- 1/2 cup almond milk
- 1 tablespoon honey

Instructions

1. Put all ingredients in a blender.
2. Blend until well mixed.
3. Pour into a glass and drizzle honey on top.

10. Green Detox Smoothie

Ingredients
- 1 cup kale
- 1/2 cucumber
- 1 green apple
- 1/2 lemon (peeled)
- 1 tablespoon spirulina powder

Instructions
1. Wash and chop all ingredients.
2. Blend until smooth.
3. Serve fresh for a detoxifying boost.

11. Mango Ginger Zinger Smoothie

Ingredients
- 1 cup mango chunks
- 1/2 inch ginger
- 1/2 cup Greek yogurt
- 1/2 cup coconut water

Instructions
1. Blend all ingredients until smooth.
2. Pour into a glass and savor the zing.

12. Blueberry Almond Bliss Smoothie

Ingredients

- 1 cup blueberries
- 1/4 cup almonds
- 1/2 banana
- 1/2 cup almond milk

Instructions

1. Put all ingredients in a blender.

2. Blend until creamy and smooth.

3. Pour into a glass and enjoy.

13. Pomegranate Paradise Smoothie

Ingredients

- 1/2 cup pomegranate seeds
- 1/2 cup strawberries
- 1/2 banana
- 1/2 cup coconut water

Instructions

1. Blend all ingredients until well combined.

2. Pour into a glass and experience paradise.

14. Cherry Vanilla Delight Smoothie

Ingredients
- 1 cup cherries (pitted)
- 1/2 cup Greek yogurt
- 1/2 banana
- 1/2 cup almond milk

Instructions
1. Blend all ingredients until smooth.
2. Pour into a glass and savor the delightful flavor.

15. Citrus Carrot Glow Juice

Ingredients
- 3 carrots
- 2 oranges
- 1/2 lemon (peeled)
- 1-inch ginger

Instructions
1. Wash and chop the carrots, oranges, lemon, and ginger.
2. Run them through a juicer.
3. Mix well and serve for a refreshing glow.

16. Cranberry Cleansing Juice

Ingredients

- 1 cup cranberries
- 2 apples
- 1 cucumber
- 1/2 lemon (peeled)

Instructions

1. Clean and cut the cranberries, apples, cucumber, and lemon.

2. Juice all ingredients together.

3. Stir and enjoy the cleansing benefits.

17. Spinach and Pineapple Power Smoothie

Ingredients

- Handful of spinach
- 1 cup pineapple chunks
- 1/2 banana
- 1/2 cup coconut water
- 1 tablespoon chia seeds

Instructions

1. Add all ingredients in a blender.

2. Blend until smooth and creamy.

3. Pour into a glass and experience the power.

18. Almond Joy Smoothie

Ingredients
- 1/4 cup almonds
- 2 tablespoons cocoa powder
- 1 banana
- 1/2 cup Greek yogurt
- 1/2 cup almond milk

Instructions
1. Blend almonds, cocoa powder, banana, Greek yogurt, and almond milk.
2. Blend until the mixture is smooth.
3. Pour into a glass for a delightful almond joy treat.

19. Orange Creamsicle Smoothie

Ingredients
- 2 oranges
- 1/2 banana
- 1/2 cup Greek yogurt
- 1/2 cup almond milk
- 1 tablespoon honey

Instructions

1. Peel and segment the oranges.

2. Blend oranges, banana, Greek yogurt, almond milk, and honey until creamy.

3. Pour into a glass for a nostalgic creamsicle flavor.

20. Peachy Protein Smoothie

Ingredients

- 1 cup frozen peaches
- 1/2 cup cottage cheese
- 1/2 banana
- 1/2 cup almond milk
- 1 tablespoon flax seeds

Instructions

1. Blend frozen peaches, cottage cheese, banana, almond milk, and flaxseeds until smooth.

2. Pour into a glass for a protein-packed peachy delight.

Conclusion

In the symphony of stroke recovery, this cookbook serves as a harmonious guide, blending the healing power of nutrition with the joy of delicious flavors. Each recipe is a note in the journey toward rejuvenation, carefully composed to nourish the body and delight the senses. As we savor the vibrant palette of ingredients, let this collection be a source of inspiration for stroke recovery seniors—a testament that wellness can be both a nourishing feast and a celebration of life.

May these culinary melodies continue to resonate, guiding you towards strength, vitality, and a flavorful chapter in the book of your recovery. Cheers to a healthier, tastier, and more harmonious tomorrow.